Head Injury Education

A Group Therapy Manual

WITHDRAWN

3 0 APR 2023

Head Injury Education

A Group Therapy Manual

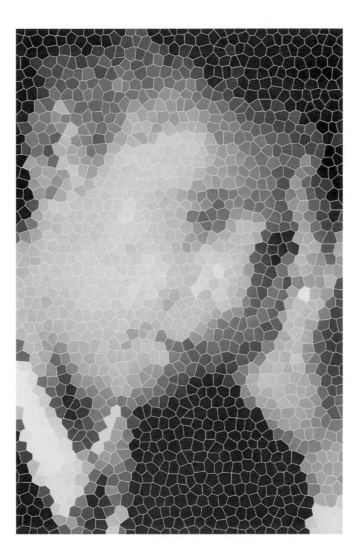

Martin van den Broek & Beverley Dayus

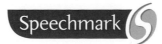

Speechmark Publishing Ltd
Telford Road, Bicester, Oxon OX26 4LQ, UK

First published in 2002 by
Speechmark Publishing Ltd, Telford Road, Bicester, Oxon OX26 4LQ, UK

www.speechmark.net

002-4213/Printed in the United Kingdom/1030

British Library Cataloguing in Publication Data

Broek, M D van den, 1959–
    Head injury education: a group therapy manual
    1. Head – Wounds and injuries – Patients – Rehabilitation
    2. Group psychotherapy
    I. Title   II. Dayus, Beverley
    617.4'81'06516

ISBN 0 86388 229 3

Contents

Forms

Overheads

Handouts

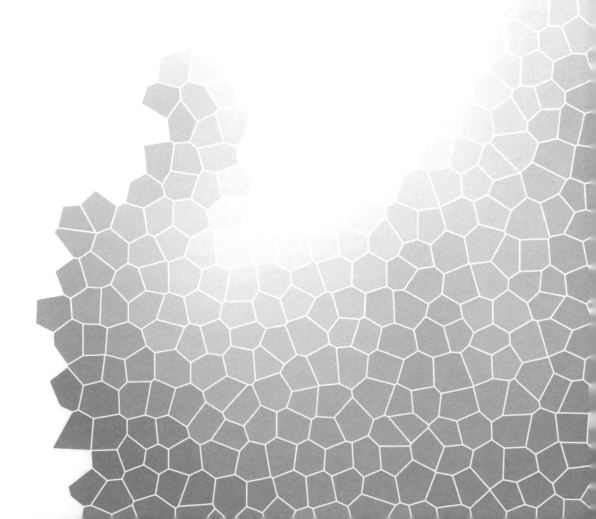

Section 1

Introduction

The Head Injury Education (HIE) group was designed to be one component of a post-acute neuropsychologically-oriented rehabilitation programme for patients with acquired brain injuries. Post-acute programmes commonly have several components, including cognitive rehabilitation; individual and group therapy; and family and social interventions (Ben-Yishay, 1996; Prigatano, 1997). Typically, they also include sessions aimed at educating participants about the effects of brain injuries (eg, Wesolowski & Zencius, 1994). This manual outlines a group therapy programme designed for patients with traumatic brain injuries (TBI), although with modifications it could include those who have other conditions, such as strokes, neoplasms and infections.

The HIE manual sets out the reasoning behind the programme, as well as providing the material needed to carry out the sessions. Although the session plans are intended to be self-explanatory, and in many respects the material is straightforward, in practice the group can elicit issues and concerns among the participants that require skilled responses from the treating therapists. For this reason, it is essential that those running the group are experienced in brain injury rehabilitation, as well as familiar with the complexities of group and individual therapy.

The first section of the manual reviews some of the relevant background knowledge for implementing the group, including the causes and consequences of TBI, and the rehabilitation process. Practical guidelines and suggestions for practice are given, and the problem of impaired insight is discussed. Section 2 describes the programme, and includes an outline of the aims of each session, its structure and the necessary materials.

Aims of the Head Injury Education group

Although educational interventions can be useful at any time after TBI, the HIE group was developed for those who are past the acute phase of their rehabilitation, when the primary concern of treatment is the patient's medical and physical condition. In practice, this is usually at least some months after the injury, when the focus of rehabilitation turns to the future, and community reintegration.

The aims of the HIE group are threefold. First, at a basic level the sessions are meant to help participants to understand and learn about the effects of TBI. It is a common clinical observation that many survivors of a TBI are keen to understand and make sense of their experiences. TBI is nearly always a sudden and unexpected event, following a motor vehicle crash, fall or assault; therefore, the survivor will have undergone an abrupt transition from their premorbid state to a life of disability. As a result, many people require clear, impartial information and advice about the injuries they have sustained; guidance on strategies to ameliorate those difficulties, and the opportunity to discuss the future. Regrettably, it is also a common observation that many TBI survivors have difficulty obtaining this information. Therefore, the aim of the HIE group is to fill this gap. Within the group, the TBI participants are called *trainees* and the therapists are called *trainers*, to reflect the educational as opposed to the clinical spirit of the sessions. As the amount and variety of information that trainees require is potentially vast, only the more common problems after TBI have been included. However, although the group is educational in orientation, it should not be run in a didactic manner. As a rule, the sessions work best if the trainers are able to establish an informal, interactive style, and pace the amount and complexity of the material to the needs and abilities of the individual trainees, allowing ample opportunity for discussion and questions.

Second, the sessions are intended to help raise insight and self-awareness. The degree to which an individual retains their self-awareness is an important predictor of their likely response to rehabilitation (Prigatano, 1991, 1997; Sherer *et al*, 1998). Poor insight may be due to the insult to the brain; it may arise as a defence mechanism in response to the injuries sustained, or it may be a combination of the two. In any event, the effect is the same: namely, poor engagement in rehabilitation for deficits that are not recognised or seen as significant. Attempts to raise self-awareness can be fraught with problems, and may bring about only acquiescence with the rehabilitation process. On occasion, attempting to raise insight in too confrontational a manner can be counterproductive, and may precipitate despondency or resistance. The approach taken in the HIE group is not to address trainees' self-awareness directly, as this can be threatening, especially in a group setting. Instead, the focus is on reviewing the range of problems that potentially can arise following trauma. The process of reviewing difficulties is intended to encourage self-reflection and comparison. Moreover, the group format allows individuals to listen to the problems and experiences of other trainees within a supportive milieu, and this can be an additional powerful mechanism for self-appraisal. Finally, an important technique used throughout the sessions is the role-reversal procedure in the case analyses. This involves trainees in reviewing a case study of a head-injured person; taking on the role of the person's therapist and making recommendations to overcome their difficulties. The exercises are intended to encourage trainees to reflect on their own difficulties in a non-threatening manner, and in practice most people find them both novel and enjoyable.

Third, the HIE group is intended to build motivation. Variable and poor motivation for change is not uncommon among those engaged in rehabilitation. It is well established that gains from post-acute rehabilitation can be modest, and may fail to generalise or be maintained in the long term (Wesolowski & Zencius, 1994; Sohlberg & Raskin, 1996). The causes of such problems are multifaceted, and one important factor is limited or fluctuating motivation on the part of the TBI survivor. Throughout the HIE sessions, trainees are provided with information, and the opportunity to discuss issues of concern. However, much time is also spent reviewing strategies that trainees can employ themselves to overcome or ameliorate their disabilities. While ventilation is an appropriate function of the HIE group, trainers should be alert to the possibility of a particular session or sessions becoming merely a forum for the repetition of problems, without consideration of the steps that might improve a trainee's situation. The intention is to educate trainees to recognise that relatively modest changes may bring about significant improvements, and so enhance self-efficacy. Although the sessions address issues such as compensatory memory aids and overcoming emotional problems, it is not intended that the group should be the primary means of rehabilitating these difficulties. The HIE group is nearly always one of a number of therapeutic groups and individual sessions, which may include a memory group, attention retraining, and so on. However, the HIE sessions are intended to reinforce and build motivation to engage appropriately with these sessions.

Although throughout the programme a good deal of information is imparted, the final two sessions differ from what has gone before, and require trainees to complete personal presentations. These involve each trainee presenting themselves to the group. To facilitate this process, trainees are asked to complete a form that reviews their various problems, and involves clarifying the practical steps they intend to take to overcome their difficulties. The exercise requires trainees to draw on previous HIE sessions and other rehabilitation groups, and individual work. Most importantly, it is intended to help trainees focus upon those strategies that will be of use to them, and formally confirm and commit to their personal rehabilitation plan.

Post-acute neurorehabilitation

During the last 20 years there has been an explosion of interest in the development of post-acute brain injury rehabilitation programmes (van den Broek, 1999). The HIE group was developed as a weekly session in a programme that trainees attended two days a week for 12 weeks. The trainers were drawn from a number of disciplines, including neuropsychology, therapy professions, nursing and nursing assistants. The programme consisted of the following components:

Community meeting: Each week trainees and trainers met together to discuss the programme; problems that had arisen, and trainees' progress. During the programme, trainees were asked to prepare a presentation each on an issue of interest to themselves and the group. These included talks on the effects of alcohol and TBI; epilepsy; memory aids, and so on. Guest speakers were also invited to the meeting to talk about issues of interest: for example, state benefits; support services in the community, and educational opportunities.

Memory strategies group: The memory group introduced compensatory strategies to reduce limitations due to amnesia. The group followed the three-stage model of memory rehabilitation developed by Sohlberg *et al* (1994), and involved awareness training; instruction in the use of compensatory aids, and generalisation training.

Problem-solving training: The problem-solving group provided instruction in problem recognition; goal definition; consequential and means-end thinking, and decision-making.

Social skills training: This group involved training in the use and recognition of both verbal and non-verbal communication skills. Role-play exercises were used throughout, and some sessions were videotaped for group and individual feedback.

Living skills: Following occupational therapy assessment, trainees were seen for training in activities of daily living such as cooking, shopping, and community mobility, either within the rehabilitation facility or in the community.

Attention retraining: Each trainee received regular individual sessions of attention process training (Sohlberg & Mateer, 1987), focused on enhancing attentional skills such as sustained, selective and alternating attention.

Individual sessions: In addition to the group sessions, trainees were seen individually by a designated keyworker to discuss personal issues; review progress on the programme, and check up on assignments. Family members were encouraged to attend to familiarise themselves with the programme and the tasks for completion at home. Progress on the programme was monitored by scaling trainees' individual goals within a goal attainment scaling format (Tobbell & Burns, 1997).

Characteristics of traumatic brain injury

Head injury has been called the 'silent epidemic', with many survivors and little representation. The overall annual incidence is estimated to be in the order of 300 per 100,000, although there are considerable difficulties in determining the true numbers, and there is substantial regional variation (British Society of Rehabilitation Medicine, 1998). The majority of people who have a head injury are young males who have sustained their injuries due to a road traffic accident. A high proportion of those who have serious injuries become unemployed; have difficulty re-establishing social relationships, and represent a significant stress upon their families and carers (Brooks *et al*, 1987a, 1987b; Ponsford, 1995). Cognitive impairments such as forgetfulness; loss of concentration, and poor planning and organisational skills are common, as well as emotional problems such as depression, irritability, and anxiety (Ponsford, 1995).

Traumatic injuries can be classified as being either 'penetrating' or 'closed'. A penetrating (or 'open') head injury results from an object entering the skull and brain – for example, from a gunshot injury. Penetrating injuries tend to have more localised effects than closed injuries, and lead to more discreet impairments. A closed head injury occurs when the head is hit, banged, or badly shaken, but the skull is not penetrated – for example, in the course of a car accident or fall. The brain may suffer contusions (bruising) and diffuse axonal injury. It may be damaged at the site of contact (a coup injury), and then rebound and damage the opposite side (a contrecoup injury). As the brain is shaken, it can be torn by small, bony protrusions from the skull. Certain areas have bony ridges that increase the likelihood of damage, most notably in the frontal and temporal regions. Further cerebral injury may occur due to secondary complications, including disruption of the oxygen supply to the brain; bleeding within the skull, or the development of infections such as meningitis.

The problems that result from TBI are many and varied. Most people make a good physical recovery, whereas many have enduring cognitive, emotional and behavioural problems. Although a wide range of cognitive problems is found, in practice memory, attention and dysexecutive impairments often represent the primary obstacles to community reintegration and employment (van den Broek, 1999). Therefore, these problems have been selected for review and discussion in the HIE programme, and trainees are encouraged to consider strategies to ameliorate their effects. Emotional problems after TBI range from aggression and anger through to depression, apathy, and emotional lability. Their causes are often multifaceted, and include the severity and site of the brain damage; self-appraisal; the reactions of others; and the influence of social problems such as unemployment, financial difficulties; and inactivity. Trainees are encouraged to review these problems and consider their potential causes, both through the case analyses and their own experiences.

Lack of insight can take many forms, ranging from frank denial of impairments through to a tendency to minimise the significance of problems (Giacino & Cicerone, 1998). Impaired awareness has been identified as an important determinant of outcome for brain-injured patients (Prigatano, 1991; Prigatano & Weinstein, 1996; Sherer *et al*, 1998). For this reason, many therapists view raising insight as an important goal, so as to engage the survivor in rehabilitation. This may not be without its problems, however, as raised insight can be associated with anxiety and depression. As awareness of deficits increases, a person's self-image may decrease: having denied or minimised the effects of a head injury, the realisation of disability may precipitate distress. It is important that this process is directed towards acceptance and adjustment, and is not inadvertently neglected by the treating team. Thus HIE trainers must observe carefully individuals within the group, and be prepared to deal with any emotional disturbance that develops.

Group therapy in neurorehabilitation

Group therapy has a relatively short history in brain-injury rehabilitation, although its advantages have been expounded by a number of practitioners, and are now well known (Christensen *et al*, 1996; Ben-Yishay, 1996). It is thought that TBI survivors gain greater understanding of their problems in a milieu that is understanding and supportive. It has been suggested that a key component is that participants are no longer viewed as 'patients', but as individual citizens and members of families (Ben-Yishay, 1996). Talking and listening to people with similar difficulties, and sharing coping strategies, are considered important elements in instilling hope and optimism.

By pooling experiences and listening to others, trainees may reduce feelings of isolation while learning to recognise their own problems. Feedback from other group members can convey therapeutic messages that might be rejected by a trainee in more formal treatment encounters with rehabilitation staff. Inappropriate behaviours and statements may be modified in response to the reactions of group members, who may shape more appropriate social skills. The process of helping each other may have the invaluable effect of enhancing a trainee's self-image. As well as these therapeutic benefits, there are also significant practical advantages in utilising group approaches – one of the most important being that they address the needs of several people simultaneously, and therefore represent an efficient use of therapists' time and resources.

Organisational and practical issues

When establishing an education group, it is important to bear in mind some of the following issues:

Trainee selection: The HIE group was designed primarily for people who have sustained a TBI. However, those who have suffered other non-degenerative brain disorders, such as encephalitis or anoxia, may readily be included following amendments to some of the sessions. A more important consideration is that the group should be closed, and that only trainees who are able to commit to the full programme are selected. Variable attendance, or a drop-out of trainees, invariably has a corrosive effect on the group atmosphere, and substantially undermines the gains derived by the remaining trainees. The content is intended to build understanding cumulatively, with each session developing upon the previous week, and it is therefore important that all the sessions are attended.

Group size: About eight trainees seems to be the optimum group size. Such a group is small enough to allow a degree of integration, but sufficiently large to allow the formation of smaller groups for the case analyses.

Session length: Each session is intended to last an hour, although – depending on the capabilities of the trainees – sessions of an hour and a half may be appropriate. Many TBI survivors have limited attention and fatigue easily, so trainers must monitor the tolerance of the group carefully, and adjust their approach accordingly. As might be expected, some trainees have no difficulty tolerating the amount of material covered, and indeed they may find it insufficient for their needs, and require additional input, whereas others find the work taxing. Trainers should be flexible in their approach, and deal with queries and issues as they arise, at the expense of covering all the material suggested. For some trainees, the session guidelines may contain too much material, or alternatively, it may be beneficial to review previous sessions at length to ensure understanding. Material can be modified, omitted or carried over from one session to another as seems appropriate. Trainers should be prepared to digress from the session outlines as issues of interest are raised, and they should not stick rigidly to the proposed format.

Leadership of sessions: Usually two trainers are needed to run the group, with one taking the lead role of introducing the session material. The second trainer has a key role in providing support – for instance, in answering difficult questions; facilitating the small group exercises, and helping trainees prepare their personal presentations. Not surprisingly, a relaxed, informal style among the trainers makes for a more successful group, and despite the sessions' educational nature, it is important that trainers avoid falling into the trap of presenting themselves as experts.

Materials: Each session requires certain materials. It can be helpful for those trainees who have significant memory problems if each trainee is photographed at the beginning of the programme, and their picture and name posted on a board. Trainees should be issued with a folder in which to store course handouts and personal notes. In some sessions, trainees are provided with handouts for home reading, and it is important that in the following week there is a review of the material to monitor understanding. In all sessions, the equipment needed includes a white-board, flip-chart paper, felt-tip pens and an overhead projector. For some of the sessions it may also be helpful to have a model brain and skull as teaching aids.

Location: A spacious room is required, in which the chairs are organised in a circular fashion to create an informal and relaxed atmosphere. The trainers should not sit together. The room should have enough space so that the participants can move around easily and break into smaller groups.

Group policy: It may be helpful – and, on occasion, essential – to have the group draw up a list of rules by which it operates. These may cover issues such as non-attendance; interruptions and turn-taking; use of sexist language; breaks, and so on. Such policies can be important for the cohesion of the group, as they set the ground rules by which trainees engage with one another, and they can be cited if infractions occur. The rules should be developed collectively, so that each trainee shares their ownership, and they should be written up and posted in the therapy room.

Monitoring progress

It is a growing requirement of those working in neurorehabilitation that they audit their work, and are able to demonstrate the effectiveness of their interventions (McMillan & Sparkes, 1999). Unfortunately, however, there is as yet no consensus as to the measures that should be used to demonstrate clinical outcomes, and, in particular, no method of demonstrating the utility of educational programmes. Progress in the HIE group can be monitored qualitatively: for instance, trainees may report that the opportunity to talk to trainers and other trainees; ventilate and share experiences; and explore solutions are valuable benefits. Such accounts are important, and may be associated with real clinical change, although necessarily they are subjective and non-empirical. Trainers may wish to develop scholastic-type tests – for instance, of trainees' knowledge of anatomy, and the effects of TBI – which can be administered before and after the sessions (see Wesolowski & Zencius, 1994).

One approach that lends itself particularly well to assessing the effectiveness of the group is the 'question and answer' method described by Sohlberg *et al* (1994). This technique was developed to raise insight, and assess the effectiveness of memory rehabilitation. The therapist draws up a list of 10 questions to ask the TBI survivor about their memory problems and memory systems: for instance, in what way their memory has been affected; how they would use a memory aid to deal with an everyday problem, and so on. Different questions are developed for different TBI survivors, according to their individual needs and limitations. Trainees' responses are scored according to the degree of assistance they require in providing the answers. If the trainee cannot recall the information, and the trainer has to provide the answer, a score of 2 is awarded; a verbal prompt or cue scores 1; if the trainee spontaneously provides the correct answer, the score is zero. High overall scores therefore indicate a high degree of prompting and difficulty in spontaneously recalling answers. By repeating the procedure at different intervals, the therapist can monitor change over time. The same method can be used with little modification to assess trainees' understanding and retention of information on the HIE course.

For each session, a checklist and progress form is provided, which trainers can use to record the material covered; assess issues that have arisen, such as the suitability of the material; and summarise each trainee's response to the session. The forms are intended to be used by trainers to reflect on the impact of each session, so that they can adjust and tailor their approach flexibly throughout the course.

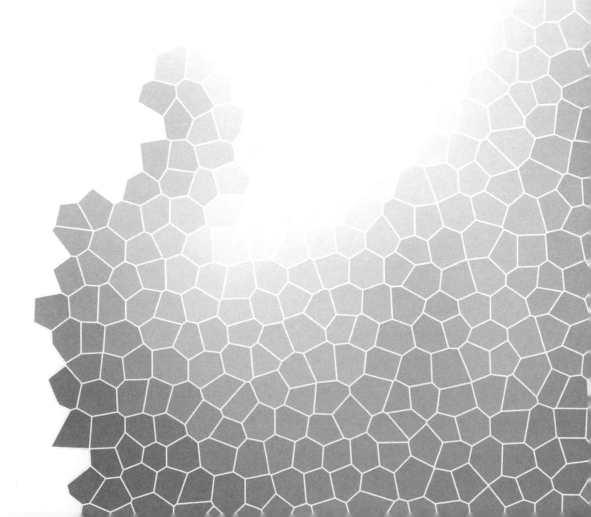

Section 2

Session 1

TOPICS
Aims of the session
Personal introductions
Session outline
Aims of the course
Characteristics of TBI
Types and severity of TBI

Aims of the session

> 1 **Introduce trainees to the other group members and trainers.**
> 2 **Outline the aims of the HIE group.**
> 3 **Provide a general introduction to the causes of TBI.**

Personal introductions

The session begins with introductions from the trainers, and an exercise to introduce each of the trainees. This can be done by suggesting that each trainee turns to the person sitting on their left and ask their name; brief details about their injury (such as how long since their TBI, how it was sustained); in what way they hope to benefit by being in the group; and any other personal details (such as hobbies or interests). Trainers may suggest that the trainees make a note of these details, if needed due to forgetfulness. Each trainee is then asked to introduce briefly the person they have 'interviewed' to the group.

The trainers can then address any housekeeping issues (such as availability of coffee/tea, smoking areas, toilets), and hand out folders for the course material.

Session outline

The lead trainer starts by saying that a common complaint of people who have had a TBI is that, although their acute medical care was very satisfactory,

14

nevertheless, they have never had the opportunity to discuss properly what has happened to them, and to make sense of their symptoms and difficulties. This may be because medical staff are often busy and lack time to discuss such issues, or because they do not always have a good understanding of the long-term effects of brain injury.

Aims of the course

The aims of the course are then written on a flip-chart, or presented using an overhead projector (Overhead 1.1):

> **1 To provide information on the nature and consequences of traumatic brain injury (TBI).**
> **2 To outline methods to overcome the effects of TBI.**

Trainees should be encouraged to volunteer their experiences of their acute care, and the degree to which they, their relatives and professionals understand TBI. It should be stressed that a central aim of the course is to provide the opportunity for trainees to ask about problems and how they might be overcome, and they should feel free to ask questions and make notes as required.

Characteristics of TBI

The lead trainer then introduces the initial topics for the session – an outline of the incidence and causes of head injury. The material may be introduced in the form of a series of questions using an overhead (Overhead 1.2), or by writing the questions on a flip-chart. Trainees are asked to estimate the incidence each year, and, if local figures are available, they can be asked to estimate the annual numbers in the area served by the rehabilitation service. It can be emphasised that TBI is a common, although often unrecognised and relatively poorly understood, condition. Questions include the following:

How many people have a TBI each year?
What are the most common causes of TBI?
Who has a TBI?

15

The same questioning method can be used to introduce the causes of TBI, and to identify who is at risk. Attention can be drawn to any similarities that exist between these details and the composition of the group.

Types and severity of TBI

The trainer then introduces trainees to the different types of injury, by asking if they have come across the terms *penetrating* and *closed* head injury – perhaps in books, self-help pamphlets, or medico-legal reports. The terms can be defined using an overhead (Overhead 1.3), and the difference between them clarified. It should be emphasised that closed injuries – while superficially less serious than open injuries – can be equally, or more, disabling, depending on the severity of the impact, and the presence or lack of other complications.

Finally, the trainer introduces methods for grading the severity of TBI using the overheads *Glasgow coma scale* (Overhead 1.4) and *Post-traumatic amnesia* (Overhead 1.5). The importance of post-traumatic amnesia as a guide to the severity of the injury, and the likelihood of future cognitive, emotional and behavioural problems, are discussed. Such problems are invariably hidden, and may therefore be misunderstood. Trainees can be invited to discuss the reactions of other people – such as friends and relatives – to their difficulties. It should be stressed that, although much of what has been discussed has been relatively technical and probably unfamiliar, there will be many opportunities to go over the material again in later sessions.

Check when done

- ☐ 1 Introductions
- ☐ 2 Housekeeping issues
- ☐ 3 Aims of the course
- ☐ 4 Characteristics of TBI
- ☐ 5 Penetrating and closed TBI
- ☐ 6 Severity of TBI
- ☐ 7 Questions and answers

Session evaluation

(review issues/topics arising, type and quality of group interaction, suitability of material, topics requiring further review)

Trainees' progress

(note individual trainee's participation in session; comprehension and retention of material; emotional response to material and to other trainees; need for additional individual education or support)

Aims of the course

1 To provide information on the nature and consequences of traumatic brain injury (TBI)

2 To outline methods to overcome the effects of TBI

OVERHEAD 1.2 INTRODUCING THE MATERIAL

How many people have a TBI?

Numbers of new cases every year are estimated at 300 for every 100,000 people in the United Kingdom.

◆ These figures do not include those who have other acquired brain injuries, such as brain infections or stroke.

Brain injures have been called 'the silent epidemic'.

What causes TBI?

Road traffic accidents are responsible for approximately 70 per cent of TBIs.

Other causes include assaults, industrial accidents, falls and sporting accidents.

Who has a head injury?

Young people between 15 and 30 years.

2 to 3 males have a head injury for every female who has one.

People who are risk-takers.

People who have consumed alcohol.

Penetrating head injury

◆ Penetrating head injuries occur when the skull, and the brain within, are penetrated by an object such as a bullet or shell fragments.

Closed head injury

◆ Closed head injuries occur when the head suffers an impact, but the skull remains intact (eg, when someone is thrown about in a car accident). The head (and brain inside) suffers powerful forces of acceleration and deceleration that may cause a loss of consciousness and damage throughout the brain.

◆ The Glasgow Coma Scale is used to monitor recovery or deterioration in consciousness after a head injury.

◆ A patient's ability to open their eyes, move and speak is assessed and scored.

◆ A deterioration may mean that urgent neurosurgery is required, perhaps because of bleeding inside the skull.

Post-traumatic amnesia is the interval of time between the head injury and a person regaining day-to-day memory and being oriented to their surroundings. It includes any period of coma.

PTA	Severity
Less than 5 minutes	Very mild
5–60 minutes	Mild
1 hour–24 hours	Moderate
1–7 days	Severe
1–4 weeks	Very severe
More than 4 weeks	Extremely severe

Session 2

Aims of the session

> 1 To review the mechanisms of TBI.
> 2 To allow trainees to share their personal experiences of their injuries.

Session outline

The group begins with a review of the material covered in the previous session. If necessary, the overheads used in Session 1 should be viewed again, and clarification given on issues that arise. Trainees should be encouraged to raise queries and make notes for future reference, if required.

Mechanisms of TBI: primary and secondary injuries

The lead trainer explains the aim of the session, which is to outline how the brain is damaged in a TBI. There is an important distinction between *primary* and *secondary* injuries, and these can be defined using a flip-chart or overhead (Overhead 2.1).

When the brain is subjected to trauma in an acceleration/deceleration injury, it moves backwards and forwards and strikes the inside of the skull. Primary injuries (Overhead 2.2) are those that occur as a direct result of a blow or blows to the brain. They include *cerebral contusions* (bruising) and *diffuse axonal injury* (widespread damage throughout the brain). The difference between *coup* and *contrecoup* injuries should be explained, leading to a discussion of the frontal and temporal lobes being the most common sites of damage (as shown in Overhead 4.1). It can be useful to show trainees a model of a skull, to point out the irregularities in the surfaces around the temporal

23

and frontal regions, and their role in damaging these structures. *Diffuse axonal injury (DAI)* occurs when the axons are pulled, stretched and torn when the brain moves about in the skull. This type of injury can occur anywhere in the brain, which is why it is called a diffuse injury.

The trainer can then outline some of the factors that cause secondary damage using an overhead (Overhead 2.3) including:

Intracranial haematoma
Brain swelling
Infections
Respiratory failure

The trainer should stress the need for urgent medical intervention to prevent secondary brain damage. Some trainees may have undergone interventions such as a craniotomy or tracheostomy, or had their intracranial pressure monitored – so at this juncture, it may be appropriate to outline the purpose behind such procedures.

Finally, the trainer concludes by discussing some of the complexities surrounding the issues of injury and disability that cause confusion and misunderstanding. These will necessarily vary, depending on the concerns and interests of the group but may include:

Is it possible to have brain damage and a normal brain scan?
Can you have brain damage and be physically healthy?
Can you have brain damage and never have lost consciousness?
Is it possible to have long-standing problems after a mild TBI?

The trainer should distribute a handout (Handout 1), which summarises some of the material covered in this session. Although a good deal of factual information is imparted during the session, it is important to adjust the complexity and quantity of the material to a level appropriate to the group; to provide the opportunity for questions to clarify issues; and to allow time for the correction of any misunderstandings. Most importantly, discussion of acute care provides trainees with the opportunity to share and ventilate their own stories about the events surrounding their injury and survival, and for many this will be the most important benefit of the session.

Check when done

- [ ] 1 Recap previous session
- [ ] 2 Primary injury (contusions, DAI, coup and contrecoup injury)
- [ ] 3 Secondary injury (intracranial haematoma, swelling, infections, respiratory failure)
- [ ] 4 Questions and answers
- [ ] 5 Handout circulated (Handout 1)

Session evaluation

(review issues/topics arising, type and quality of group interaction, suitability of material, topics requiring further review)

Trainees' progress

(note individual trainee's participation in session, comprehension and retention of material; emotional response to material and to other trainees; need for additional individual education or support)

Primary damage

◆ Primary damage refers to injury inflicted to the brain by the direct effect of the impact.

Secondary damage

◆ Secondary damage refers to injury that the brain suffers due to later complications.

At the moment of impact, the brain may suffer bruising and widespread tearing or stretching of its nerve fibres.

Bruising of the brain

◆ A sudden blow can cause bruising (called *contusions*) to the brain.

◆ Damage can occur at the site of the impact (called a *coup* injury), or opposite the point of impact (called a *contrecoup* injury).

◆ Wherever the head is first struck, the most common sites of injury are the frontal and temporal lobes of the brain.

Diffuse injury to the brain

◆ Strong forces at the moment of impact may strain and tear the brain's nerve fibres (called *axons*) and cause widespread injury, which is called a *diffuse axonal injury*.

◆ Diffuse injuries are thought to be the most common causes of later psychological problems.

Secondary damage is injury to the brain caused by the development of medical complications. These include:

Bleeding

◆ A blood clot (called a *haematoma*) inside the skull, can exert pressure on the brain, and cause damage.

◆ Neurosurgery may be needed to drain the clot and stop bleeding.

Brain swelling

◆ Swelling of the brain may reduce the flow of blood and oxygen to brain cells.

Infections

◆ Germs entering the skull through a fracture may cause meningitis or abscesses.

Breathing difficulties

◆ Difficulty with breathing may reduce the supply of oxygen in the blood stream, and so to the brain.

HOW IS THE BRAIN DAMAGED IN A TRAUMATIC BRAIN INJURY?

When a person has a traumatic brain injury (TBI) – for instance, in a car accident – the brain may suffer what is called *primary* and *secondary* damage. Primary damage refers to injury caused directly by a blow or blows to the brain; secondary damage refers to injury caused by the later development of complications, such as swelling or bleeding inside the brain.

Primary damage

When the head is struck, the brain can suffer bruising, and widespread stretching and tearing of its nerve fibres.

Bruising: a sudden blow may cause the head (and the brain inside), to move backwards and forwards rapidly. As a result, the brain may strike the inside of the skull, and suffer bruising (called *contusions*). Damage can occur at the site of impact (called a *coup* injury), or to the opposite side of the brain from the point of injury (a *contrecoup* injury). No matter where the head is struck initially, the most common sites of damage are to the *frontal lobes* (located just behind the forehead) and the *temporal lobes* (located just above the ears).

Diffuse Axonal Injury: in an accident, the brain may be subjected to strong rotational forces, which strain and tear its nerve fibres – *axons*. This may cause the person to lapse into a coma, and may result in widespread damage – a *diffuse axonal injury*. Diffuse injuries are thought to be one of the most common causes of later psychological problems, such as personality changes, and poor memory and concentration.

Secondary Damage

Medical complications following an injury can cause additional damage, called *secondary damage*. Some of the more common complications are:

Bleeding: bleeding inside the skull can result in the development of a blood clot (*haematoma*). As the skull is rigid, the presence of a clot compresses the brain and can lead to a deterioration in a person's level of consciousness, and eventually to coma. Bleeding may occur outside or inside the brain, and depending on its degree, urgent neurosurgery may be required to drain the blood and stop further bleeding.

Brain swelling: after a TBI, swelling can occur throughout the brain, or just in a local area. In the same way that a clot compresses the brain, so swelling causes a rise in pressure inside the head, reducing the flow of blood, and so the supply of oxygen to the brain cells. When swelling is severe, doctors may insert a probe through a hole in the skull to monitor the pressure.

Infections: if the skull has been fractured, then germs may be able to enter the head and cause infection: either meningitis or pockets of infection, called abscesses.

Breathing difficulties: injuries that affect a person's ability to breathe – such as face or chest injuries – may reduce the flow of oxygen into the blood system, and so to the brain – resulting in further damage. For this reason, a person's breathing pattern is often observed carefully after a TBI and, if necessary, they may be connected to a machine called a ventilator, which assists breathing.

Session 3

Aims of the session

> **1 To understand some of the medical investigations after TBI.**
> **2 To discuss the social perceptions of TBI.**
> **3 To review the course of recovery after TBI, and the factors that contribute to its prevention.**

Session outline

As before, it is useful to start by reviewing the material discussed in the previous session, and inviting trainees to raise questions of concern. Sufficient time should be allowed for a proper discussion, addressing each issue in full before moving on to the new material.

Investigations after TBI

Usually trainees will have undergone numerous investigations during their immediate care, although their purpose may have been obscure. As the range of investigations is potentially vast, only a few can be discussed, although there should be sufficient flexibility to cover other procedures, as required. A distinction should be made between explaining the general purpose of investigations, and a trainee's personal results, which might best be discussed separately, in an individual session. The investigations are shown on an overhead (Overhead 3.1) and include:

Skull X-ray
CT brain scan
MR brain scan
EEG

Although trainees will have undergone some – or even all – of these investigations, their purpose may have been unclear. By moving through each of the assessments in turn; discussing their purpose, and addressing enquiries, the trainer should attempt to place such experiences in context. A handout that reviews these investigations (Handout 2) can be circulated to the group.

Hidden disability

Many TBI survivors have relatively few enduring physical complaints that mark them out from the general population, and this can have implications for the way they are viewed by people who are not disabled. Discussion can be cued by asking the group whether they have met with misunderstanding, or even disbelief from family, friends or statutory bodies, because they appear physically well and lack outward signs of disability. The group can be asked what difficulties this causes in terms of peoples' understanding about their individual situation, and TBI more generally. The contrast between the hidden effects of TBI and the response given to those with more overt, socially recognised signs of disability can be discussed. Finally, the group can be asked to consider what practical steps could be taken to ameliorate misunderstanding about TBI. These could include their involvement in local and national self-help groups, as well as participation in educational and other promotional initiatives.

Course of recovery after TBI

Many trainees are concerned about recovery after TBI, as a result of discussions, or what they have read in books or medico-legal reports. For some, this concern has an important bearing on their engagement in rehabilitation. The trainer introduces the topic by asking the group about their knowledge of the course of recovery after TBI. There may be considerable misconceptions – one of the most common being that once a fixed period of time has elapsed after the injury (anything ranging from six months to two years), further improvement is impossible.

It may be helpful to illustrate this model by drawing a hypothetical recovery curve on a flip-chart. This is typically negatively accelerating, up to a final level of recovery that is below a premorbid level. The trainer should introduce the idea that such curves are based on the average of group data, and do not necessarily represent the course and rate at which individual people recover. In addition, even if a person is many years post-TBI, and their neurological recovery is maximal, they can nevertheless take practical steps to improve their level of functioning and quality of life. For instance, to overcome forgetfulness they can learn to use compensatory memory aids; to cope with anxiety they can practise relaxation techniques; to deal with inactivity they can develop new roles by starting voluntary or college work, and so on. For some trainees this may be a key issue, and consequently the distinction between spontaneous neurological recovery and potential improvement through rehabilitation should be discussed fully.

Prevention of TBI

The session concludes with a group discussion about the factors that might prevent future injuries. These include:

◆ Avoiding alcohol and driving
◆ Encouraging seat-belt use
◆ Helmet use for cyclists.

As in the previous session, the amount and complexity of the material covered should be varied according to the composition of the group, and opportunity should be given for trainees to discuss their views and experiences.

Check when done

- ☐ 1 Recap previous session
- ☐ 2 Investigations after TBI
- ☐ 3 Hidden disability
- ☐ 4 Course of recovery after TBI
- ☐ 5 Prevention of TBI
- ☐ 6 Questions and answers
- ☐ 7 Handout circulated (Handout 2)

Session evaluation

(review issues/topics arising, type and quality of group interaction, suitability of material, topics requiring further review)

Trainees' progress

(note individual trainee's participation in session; comprehension and retention of material; emotional response to material and to other trainees; need for additional individual education or support)

Skull X-ray

Used to check if the skull or facial bones have been fractured.

CT (computed tomography) brain scan

Shows the brain and skull.

Reveals bruising (contusions), bleeding (haemorrhage), swelling and fractures.

MR (magnetic resonance) brain scan

Shows the brain and skull, like a CT scan.

Assesses the long-term effects of head injury.

Electroencephalography (EEG)

Records the brain's electrical activity.

Used to help diagnose epilepsy.

After TBI, a person may undergo a range of assessments and investigations, both immediately on admission to the Accident and Emergency Department, and in the weeks and months afterwards. When a person is first admitted, their blood pressure and pulse are taken, and they are examined to check their level of consciousness. The doctors will ensure that the person can breathe freely, and the pupils and limbs will be examined. Some of the more common investigations that people subsequently undergo include a skull X-ray, CT and MR brain scans, and electroencephalography.

Skull X-ray

After a TBI there may be indications – such as a leak of cerebrospinal fluid (the fluid that surrounds the brain) from an ear – that the skull has been fractured. A skull X-ray will then be taken to check whether this is the case. The presence of a fracture is important, because infection can enter the skull and, for instance, result in meningitis; there is also an increased likelihood of a blood clot developing in the brain.

CT scan

CT scans of the brain may be completed immediately after a head injury, to check whether the patient has any brain swelling, contusion or haemorrhage. Beams of X-rays are directed at the head, which allow detailed images to be taken of the entire brain. The scans can be repeated on different occasions to check on progress, and sometimes the patient is injected with a dye to obtain clear images.

MR scan

Magnetic resonance – or MR scans – tend not to be used immediately after a TBI. CT scans are used more often during the early stages of treatment. MR scans are useful for later providing detailed images of the long-term effects of the injury. They involve placing the person in a large, powerful magnet, while a computer takes images of the entire brain. As no X-rays are involved, the procedure is harmless.

Electroencephalography

An electroencephalogram – or EEG – involves placing electrodes attached to wires on to the surface of the scalp. This allows the electrical activity of the brain to be recorded. An EEG is completely harmless, and its main purpose is to help with diagnosing epilepsy. Epilepsy is repeated attacks of altered consciousness due to a disturbance of the brain's activity, and can sometimes be caused by a TBI.

Session 4

Aims of the session

> **1 To describe the frontal, temporal, parietal and occipital lobes.**
> **2 To review the functions of different brain structures.**

Session outline

As in the preceding session, it is useful to start by reviewing the material discussed previously, before moving on to the present session, which aims to describe the structure of the brain and the essential functions of each area.

Basic anatomy of the brain

The session begins with an outline of basic details about the brain – for example, that it weighs over 1 kg (about 3 lbs), and consists of between 15 and 20 billion neurons, surrounded by protective layers or membranes – meninges – and supported by cerebrospinal fluid within the skull. The trainer can indicate that the brain has many specialised areas including the *cerebrum*, *cerebellum* and *brain stem*.

Structure and functions of the frontal, temporal, parietal and occipital lobes

Using an overhead (Overhead 4.1), the trainer can show that the cerebrum consists of many folds, which have the effect of increasing its surface area. It is divided into four specialised areas: the *frontal, temporal, parietal* and *occipital lobes*. It can be helpful to point out these areas on a brain model, which is circulated for trainees to examine in more detail. The cerebrum can also be divided into two halves or *hemispheres*, and the *brainstem* and *cerebellum* should be noted, but not discussed in detail as they are reviewed in the following session.

The next step is for the trainer to outline the broad functions of each of the four lobes in turn. These can be added to the overhead, or written on a flip-chart. The material should be introduced carefully, and the complexity tailored to the abilities and interests of the group.

An overhead (Overhead 4.2) can be used to summarise the location and functions of the lobes. It should be pointed out that damage to localised areas can result in impairments in certain skills, and that the presence of these impairments is often used by clinicians such as doctors, to infer which areas of the brain have been damaged. Trainees should be reminded that the most common sites of damage after TBI are the frontal and temporal lobes, resulting in associated impairments.

Finally, the trainer provides a handout (Handout 3), which summarises these issues to aid recall.

Check when done

□ 1 Recap previous session

□ 2 Outline of anatomy of four lobes (frontal, temporal, parietal, occipital)

□ 3 Functions of the lobes

□ 4 Questions and answers

□ 5 Handout circulated (Handout 3)

Session evaluation

(review issues/topics arising, type and quality of group interaction, suitability of material, topics requiring further review)

Trainees' progress

(note individual trainee's participation in session; comprehension and retention of material; emotional response to material and to other trainees; need for additional individual education or support)

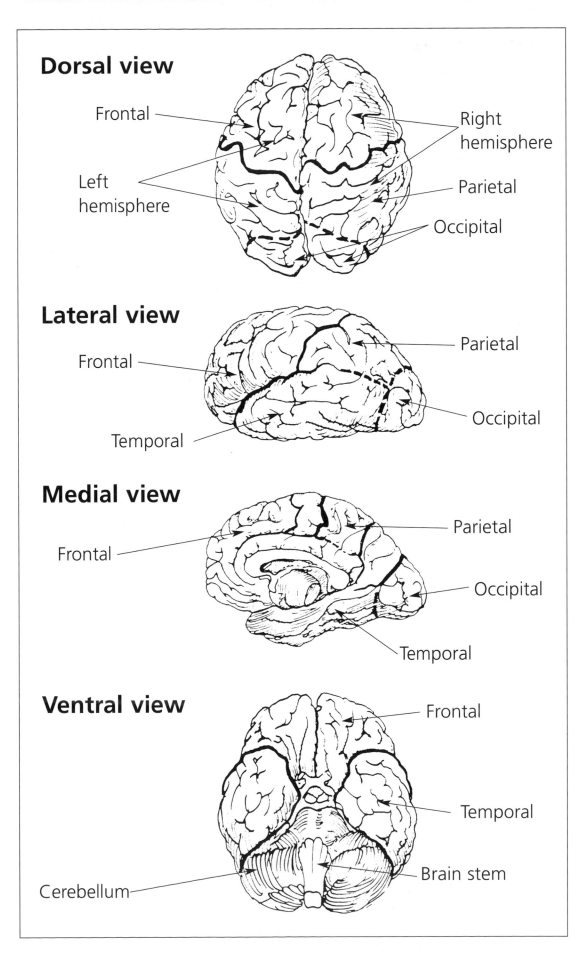

Dorsal view

Frontal

Right hemisphere

Left hemisphere

Parietal

Occipital

Lateral view

Frontal

Parietal

Temporal

Occipital

Medial view

Frontal

Parietal

Occipital

Temporal

Ventral view

Frontal

Temporal

Brain stem

Cerebellum

STRUCTURE OF THE BRAIN

Frontal lobes

- Located just behind the forehead
- Common site of injury

Important for:

- Planning
- Organisation
- Initiation
- Problem-solving and judgement
- Personality and mood
- Speech
- Movement

Parietal lobes

- Located behind the ears and towards the back of the head

Important for:

- Integrating sensory information
- Reading
- Writing
- Drawing
- Spatial judgement

Temporal lobes

- Located just above the ears
- Often damaged in head injury

Important for:

- Memory
- Hearing
- Understanding speech

Occipital lobes

- Located at the back of the head
- Uncommon site of injury

Important for:

- Vision
- Recognising objects
- Identifying colour

THE STRUCTURE OF THE BRAIN

The brain weighs over 1 kg (about 3 lbs) – approximately 2 per cent of the total body weight. It consists of billions of nerve cells that communicate with each other, so allowing the brain to process information and initiate activities.

The brain has several areas including the *cerebrum*, *cerebellum*, and the *brain stem*.

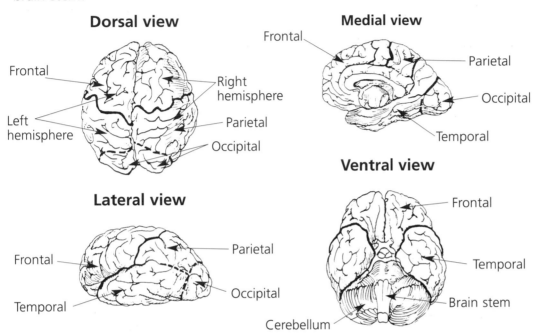

1 Cerebrum

The cerebrum accounts for most of the weight of the brain. It is covered with folds, which give it the appearance of a walnut. It has two halves (or hemispheres) and each half consists of four special areas or *lobes*, called the *frontal, temporal, parietal* and *occipital* lobes.

Frontal lobes
The frontal lobes are located behind the forehead, and they are a common site of injury after head trauma. They are known to be important areas for helping people to plan and organise themselves, initiate activities, and make judgements. In this sense they are like the chief executive of a business who plans and organises the way a company works. They are also important for speech, and damage can cause problems, ranging from a slight difficulty with finding words, to loss of the ability to speak. Frontal lobe damage can also result in personality changes and swings in mood; difficulty with problem-solving, and poor concentration. Damage may also cause a loss of or impairment to the ability to move parts of the body.

Temporal lobes
The temporal lobes are located just above the ears, and are important for hearing and understanding speech. One of the most common problems is

memory loss, and people affected have difficulty remembering conversations, events or names, although their memory for events many years ago may be relatively well preserved.

Parietal lobes

The parietal lobes are located behind the ears and towards the back of the head. They are important for integrating information from the different senses, and making sense of the information coming to the brain from the body. Problems with reading and writing may occur after parietal lobe damage, as well as difficulty with drawing or copying pictures and designs.

Occipital lobes

The occipital lobes are located at the back of the head. They have a key role in vision, and damage may result in blind spots or difficulty identifying objects or colours. As a rule, they are not a common site of damage in a head injury – the temporal and frontal lobes are affected much more often.

Left and right hemispheres

The brain consists of two halves, or hemispheres, called the left and right hemispheres. The left hemisphere is responsible for controlling movement and monitoring sensation in the right side of the body, and the right hemisphere takes on the same role for the left side. For most people, the left hemisphere is important for understanding language and speaking, as well as for other verbal skills, such as memory for conversations and written material. The right hemisphere is important for visual skills, such as drawing and copying, as well as memory for non-verbal information, such as faces.

2 Cerebellum

The cerebellum is located below the back of the cerebrum. It has a particularly important role in coordination, balance and walking. It is also important in articulation, and damage can result in slowed and slurred speech.

3 Brain stem

The brain stem connects the cerebrum with the spinal cord. It consists of a number of areas, each of which has different functions. It is important in various automatic activities, such as breathing and swallowing. Sensory messages from the body to the brain, and movement messages from the brain to the body, pass through the brain stem. It has a particular role in maintaining alertness, and damage to the brain stem can result in drowsiness.

Session 5

Aims of the session

1 **To describe the anatomy of the cerebral hemispheres, cerebellum and brain stem.**
2 **To review the functions of these structures.**

Session outline

As the trainees may have found the content of the previous session to be new and technical, it may be useful to spend some time reviewing the material and Handout 3. Following the review, the aims of this session are explained – to outline the functions of the *cerebral hemispheres, brain stem* and *cerebellum*.

Cerebral hemispheres

The trainer starts by pointing out that, as well as being differentiated into lobes, the brain is divided into two halves, or hemispheres. An overhead can be used to illustrate the anatomy (Overhead 4.1), and a brain model can be passed around the group for inspection. The trainer can introduce the idea that as well as having specialised areas (lobes), each hemisphere has different functions.

This point can be illustrated by referring to the effects of strokes on *motor functioning*. Members of the group may know of someone – perhaps a family member or friend – who has suffered a hemiparesis following a cerebrovascular accident. It can be pointed out that movement on one side of the body is controlled by the opposite, or contralateral hemisphere of the brain, which illustrates the specialised nature of the hemispheres.

The trainer then introduces the idea that cognitive abilities are also lateralised to a degree, and that for most right-handed people, their *language* abilities are located in the left hemisphere, whereas the situation is less clear-cut with left-handed people. Likewise *memory* for verbal material, such as conversations and prose, may be predominantly lateralised in the left hemisphere.

The importance of the right hemisphere in *non-verbal, visuospatial functions*, such as drawing and copying, appraising angle and music, should be discussed; as well as its role in *visual memory* for faces and designs. These distinctions are summarised on an overhead (Overhead 5.1).

It can be pointed out that damage to one hemisphere may result in relatively specific impairments. For example, discreet left-sided damage involving the temporal lobe structures may cause difficulty recalling conversations, with relative preservation of memories for non-verbal information, such as faces. Such focal damage can sometimes account for why survivors often have intact skills as well as impairments, reflecting the distribution of the brain injury sustained.

Brain stem and cerebellum

The functions of the brain stem and cerebellum can be outlined briefly using an overhead (Overhead 5.2). As the brain stem passes near bony structures, it is vulnerable to damage. Sensory information from the body to the brain, and impulses from the brain to the body, all pass through the brain stem. The trainer should review its importance in maintaining arousal and attention.

The role of the cerebellum in coordination and balance should then be discussed, as well as some of the effects of damage. These include slowness; a tendency to stagger, and slurred speech. These details are summarised in Handout 3.

For many trainees, the material covered in this and the previous session will represent their first introduction to the brain and its functions. The trainer should invite questions throughout, and utilise a brain model or other teaching aids, as appropriate. It should be stressed that the sessions are not intended to teach trainees to become neurologists, but rather to provide an overview, so that they can see that previously poorly understood symptoms have clear causes, depending on the pattern of neurological damage.

Check when done

☐ 1 Recap previous session

☐ 2 Structure and role of cerebral hemispheres

☐ 3 Structure and role of the cerebellum and brain stem

☐ 4 Questions and answers

☐ 5 Handout reviewed (Handout 3)

Session evaluation

(review issues/topics arising, type and quality of group interaction, suitability of material, topics requiring further review)

Trainees' progress

(note individual trainee's participation in session; comprehension and retention of material; emotional response to material and to other trainees; need for additional individual education or support)

OVERHEAD 5.1 THE FUNCTIONS OF THE CEREBRAL HEMISPHERES

Cerebral hemispheres

Left hemisphere	Right hemisphere
Language	Visuospatial skills
Verbal memory	Visual memory
Logical/analytical skills	Perceptual skills

OVERHEAD 5.2 THE FUNCTIONS OF THE BRAIN STEM AND CEREBELLUM

Brain stem

The brain stem is important for:

◆ Arousal and alertness

◆ Breathing

◆ Swallowing

Cerebellum

The cerebellum is important for:

◆ Coordination

◆ Balance

◆ Walking

◆ Articulation

◆ Speed of movement

Session 6

Aims of the session

Session outline

Self-assessment of memory

Case analysis: *Lucy*

Aims of the session

> **1 To understand the nature of memory impairments following TBI.**
> **2 To help trainees recognise and understand their own cognitive impairments.**

Session outline

As usual, the group begins with a review of the previous session. The trainer then explains the aims of the session, which are to understand the nature of forgetfulness, and to help trainees understand their own memory problems.

Self-assessment of memory

The trainer starts by explaining that forgetfulness is a common problem after TBI, and trainees are asked to think of examples of memory problems from their own experience. This exercise can be completed with the whole group, or alternatively trainees can be asked to write out their problems individually, using a form (Handout 4). They should include not only lapses that they have noticed, but also difficulties that relatives, carers or professionals have mentioned, or problems they have experienced when taking neuropsychological tests.

These examples are then written on a flip-chart labelled 'Memory Problems', in the order in which they are introduced. This may result in a lengthy list, which allows trainees to share their difficulties, and to become aware that others have more or less severe problems. The trainer should facilitate this pooling of experience, and point out the similarities and differences between trainees. Discrepancies between how trainees view their memory, and the feedback they have received from others, should be explored. It can be pointed out that some people are not fully aware of the problems they experience, and that this lack of insight may be another consequence of brain injury.

The next step is for the trainer to help trainees to organise these lapses under different headings:

Post-traumatic amnesia
Retrograde amnesia
Anterograde amnesia
Prospective memory loss

Each term should be defined briefly, and a definition written on a flip-chart. For instance, prospective memory loss may be defined as 'difficulty remembering future events and intentions'. Trainees may be more familiar with colloquial terms such as *long-term memory (LTM) loss* instead of *retrograde amnesia*, and *short-term memory (STM) loss*, instead of *anterograde amnesia*, and it may be more appropriate to use these labels. Trainees can be encouraged to consider which problems are the most significant for them, and interfere the most with everyday living.

Case analysis: *Lucy*

The group is then introduced to the case of *Lucy* (Handout 5). Copies of the Lucy handout are circulated to each trainee, and a volunteer is asked to read it aloud. The trainer states that Lucy has a number of cognitive problems, and asks the trainees to imagine that they are Lucy's therapist or doctor, responsible for her rehabilitation. They have to answer each of the five questions on the handout, drawing on what they have learned in this and other rehabilitation groups.

The trainees are then divided into two or three smaller groups, and provided with pens and flip-chart paper. They are asked to list the questions, and write down their answers for feedback to the full group at the end of the session. Each of the smaller groups is assigned a trainer who acts as a facilitator. A key part of the exercise is the final question, and trainees should be asked to brainstorm ideas that might help Lucy to overcome her cognitive problems, drawing on the material and ideas discussed in individual treatment sessions, and other groups and sources. The facilitator should focus the group on Lucy's case, and keep the trainees in the role of therapist, so that each of the questions is addressed as fully as possible. Form 6.1 is a sample of a completed flip-chart.

Following the feedback to the whole group, the trainees can be asked to consider whether Lucy's situation would be improved if she followed their recommendations, and what outstanding problems remain. The intention is to help trainees to begin to relate what may have seemed academic factual knowledge to real problems, and to become aware that many difficulties can be ameliorated, using relatively straightforward compensatory strategies.

The material covered in the session is summarised in Handout 6, which is circulated at the end of the session.

Check when done

☐ 1 Recap previous session

☐ 2 Trainee's self-assessment of memory problems

☐ 3 Types of memory difficulties (post-traumatic amnesia, retrograde amnesia, anterograde amnesia, prospective memory loss)

☐ 4 Case analysis: *Lucy*

☐ 5 Questions and answers

☐ 6 Handouts circulated (Handouts 4–6)

Session evaluation

(review issues/topics arising, type and quality of group interaction, suitability of material, topics requiring further review)

Trainees' progress

(note individual trainee's participation in session; comprehension and retention of material; emotional response to material and to other trainees; need for additional individual education or support)

MEMORY PROBLEMS: SELF-ASSESSMENT

In the space below, list the different kinds of memory problems you have experienced since your head injury (eg, forgetting what you did yesterday; having difficulty recalling messages; things-to-do; appointments, etc).

CASE STUDY: LUCY

Lucy, a 28-year-old mother of three young children, was a passenger in a car that was involved in an accident. She was in a coma for several hours, and then confused and disoriented for about two days. X-rays of the skull showed no fractures. Lucy was in hospital for several weeks before she went home to her family.

After her in-patient rehabilitation, Lucy expected to resume running the household as she had before. However, she found that she had difficulty remembering what she called 'silly things', such as preparing her children's packed lunches for school, or their games kit. When the teachers asked after her when she missed a Parents' Evening, she appeared confused and said she knew nothing about the meeting. She forgot appointments with the family doctor, and arrangements to meet people, and she had difficulty recalling what she wanted in shops. Sometimes she forgot things without realising it. In contrast, she seemed to remember events before the accident quite well.

Lucy's partner suggested that she should keep a notepad and write down things, but she felt this might hamper her recovery and make her dependent. She said she wanted to use her memory as much as possible to aid her recovery.

What are…

◆ *The key difficulties Lucy is experiencing?*
◆ *The effects on her daily life?*
◆ *The potential causes of her problems?*
◆ *The factors that make her situation more difficult?*
◆ *The factors that would help her handle the situation better?*

CASE ANALYSIS: LUCY

What are...

The key difficulties Lucy is experiencing?

Short-term memory loss

Can't remember appointments (prospective memory)

Her past recall (retrograde memory) is relatively good

The effects on her daily life?

Can't remember small things, eg, children's clothes, meetings, appointments

The potential causes of her problems?

Severe closed head injury — several hours' coma, PTA lasted two days, although she had no skull fracture

The factors that make her situation more difficult?

Expects to return to normal straightaway, seems impatient

Won't use a notepad; thinks it will slow her recovery

Doesn't seem to be fully aware how bad her memory is

The factors that would help her handle the situation better?

She could use memory aids, eg, notepad, diary, personal organiser

She could keep 'To-Do' lists for the children's tasks

Needs to learn about head injury — do some reading — to become more aware of her problems

Join a support group and meet other head-injured people

Change her expectations of herself

Discuss her problems with her partner and the teachers

Memory problems are common after head injury, although people differ considerably as to the type and severity of difficulties they experience. Immediately after a head injury there is often a period of confusion and disorientation which can last anywhere between minutes and several months before clearing. This period is called *post-traumatic amnesia*, or *PTA*, and as a rule of thumb the longer someone is in post-traumatic amnesia, the more severe the head injury is likely to have been.

After the post-traumatic amnesia has settled, it becomes clear whether there are more enduring memory problems. Often a person has difficulty recalling events prior to the head injury; this is called *retrograde amnesia* or *long-term memory loss*. Retrograde amnesia can stretch back for between days and months, although even after a severe injury it may be only minutes in duration.

If the injury has been serious, there is commonly a tendency to forget day-to-day events or issues, such as conversations, messages or future appointments. This forgetfulness is called *short-term memory loss* or *anterograde amnesia*. Sometimes a distinction is made between being able to remember things from the past – *retrospective memory* – and events or things that have to be done in the future – *prospective memory*. Remembering to return a telephone call later on in the day, or remembering to go to a doctor's appointment in a few days, are examples of when prospective memory is used.

Psychologists sometimes divide learning into *encoding*, *retention* and *retrieval*. *Encoding* refers to the stage of putting information into the memory store. A problem at this point, for instance, will result in limited information being placed in memory. Often, fluctuating attention is the cause of poor encoding. One way around this is to practise pacing learning on a regular basis, rather than trying to learn or study for lengthy periods. Checking that material is understood and makes sense can also help. If the information is organised in some way it is more likely to stick in memory. For instance, instead of trying to learn a long shopping list, it may be better to group the individual items under different headings, such as 'groceries' or 'toiletries'.

A problem at the *retention* stage means that once information is in store, it nevertheless fades away more rapidly than is normal. If this is the problem, then rehearsing the information and checking it is still in memory after a delay can be useful.

A problem with *retrieval* means that although information may have been properly encoded and retained over an interval, it is nevertheless difficult to get it out of the store. Most people have had the experience of not being able to remember something, and then a brief prompt or reminder causes it to flood back into memory. In this situation, the problem is retrieving the information. People with this kind of difficulty can benefit from cues or prompts; for instance, the initial letters of a name may cue retrieval of a person's full name.

Many people do not just suffer from forgetfulness. They have other problems, perhaps affecting their concentration, perceptual skills, or speech. One difficulty may be that people are not completely aware of the degree to which they have changed as a result of their head injury. For instance, someone may know that they are forgetful, but underestimate how often they forget or mislay things, or ask questions without realising that they have already been answered. In extreme cases, someone may deny that they have any problems, whereas a relative will say that they are extremely forgetful. Limited awareness makes it difficult to overcome forgetfulness, as people are unlikely to use a memory aid such as a diary effectively, if they do not think they have much of a problem. In this situation, feedback from other people – such as relatives, friends and professional staff – can be helpful in clarifying what kind of memory problems are present, and their severity.

Session 7

Aims of the session

1 To understand the different kinds of problems with attention that occur after TBI.

2 To help trainees to understand and recognise their own cognitive impairments.

Session outline

The trainer starts by discussing how poor attention and concentration can result in apparent forgetfulness, not because the head-injured person has necessarily forgotten information, but because it was not properly learned (or encoded) in the first place. This leads to a review of the different kinds of attentional impairments, and the following terms can be introduced and explained:

Sustained attention
Selective attention
Divided attention

Self-assessment of attention

Using an overhead (Overhead 7.1), the trainer can illustrate examples of the different types of problems. Each member of the group is then given a self-rating sheet, Handout 7. They are asked to list briefly practical examples of any attentional problems they have experienced since their injury, and to illustrate the degree to which they interfere with everyday life. These problems are then fed back to the whole group, who confirm the categorisation on a flip-chart. Many problems will not differ substantially from those that trainees experienced pre-injury: the main differences will be in the frequency and severity of the lapses. This can also be discussed.

Overcoming attentional difficulties

The next step is an individual exercise in which each trainee brainstorms ideas that might overcome these difficulties. It may be necessary for the trainer to provide examples to start the process, and some trainees may require individual assistance to complete the exercise. The ideas of the entire group are then written on a flip-chart and, if successful, the exercise should result in a lengthy list including ideas such as:

> *Work or read for short periods*
> *Take frequent rests or breaks*
> *Only study when refreshed*
> *Avoid noisy environments*
> *Practise relaxation and breathing exercises*
> *Use memory aids (eg, diary)*
> *Monitor my mood for feelings of irritation*
> *Avoid alcohol, drugs*
> *Complete complex tasks when rested (eg, morning), and easy tasks later*
> *Practise and repeat when learning*
> *Change activities frequently to avoid getting bored*
> *Keep a check (self-monitor) on attention-span*
> *Learn in quiet, stress-free places*
> *Avoid tight deadlines*

The aim of this exercise is to illustrate that simple strategies, such as self-pacing or avoiding noise, can have a significant beneficial effect, and minimise the impact of underlying attentional difficulties. Finally, the trainer can ask trainees to consider which strategy or strategies would be most helpful to them, and how they might incorporate their use into their daily routine.

Trainees can be asked to consider what advantages they would derive if they used any of the strategies, and what practical steps they would have to take to implement them. The session concludes with the trainer circulating Handout 8 that summarises the material covered in the session.

Check when done

☐ 1 Recap previous session

☐ 2 Types of attentional difficulties (sustained, selective and divided attention)

☐ 3 Trainee's self-assessment of attentional problems

☐ 4 Overcoming attentional problems: individual and group exercise

☐ 5 Questions and answers

☐ 6 Handouts circulated (Handouts 7 and 8)

Session evaluation

(review issues/topics arising, type and quality of group interaction, suitability of material, topics requiring further review)

Trainees' progress

(note individual trainee's participation in session; comprehension and retention of material; emotional response to material and to other trainees; need for additional individual education or support)

Sustained attention

Problems with sustained attention occur when someone has difficulty concentrating on the same thing for prolonged periods:

◆ 'My mind wanders when I try to read.'

◆ 'I can't watch a film the whole way through.'

Selective attention

Poor selective attention refers to having difficulty concentrating on one task, and ignoring distractions:

  'I can't concentrate on my coursework if there are noises in the house.'

  'I can't follow what someone is saying in a crowded pub.'

Divided attention

Difficulty with divided attention occurs when someone finds it hard to do two or more things at the same time:

  'I can't keep my mind on the cooking if someone talks to me.'

  'I can't take in what the teacher is saying and make notes at the same time.'

PROBLEMS WITH ATTENTION: SELF-ASSESSMENT

In the space below, list briefly examples of some of the different kinds of concentration problems you have experienced since your injury.

Sustained attention problems *(difficulty concentrating for prolonged periods)*:

Selective attention problems *(difficulty ignoring distractions)*:

Divided attention problems *(difficulty completing two or more tasks at the same time)*:

CONCENTRATION DIFFICULTIES

Problems with concentration and attention are common after a head injury, and may result in difficulties following conversations or attending to a book. Sometimes these difficulties are very marked: people are unable to stick to a task for long, or they are easily distracted. However, even minor lapses can be quite disabling in certain circumstances; they could, for example, stop a surgeon or airline pilot working. Attentional problems can take different forms, such as having difficulty reading for long periods; being unable to deal with more than one thing at a time, or being easily distracted.

Sustained attention

'My mind wanders when I try to read.'
'I can't watch a film the whole way
through without getting up.'

Some people have difficulty with what is called sustained attention. This means that although they are able to complete a task such as reading, or working on a piece of equipment, they have difficulty sustaining themselves on activities for long periods. For instance, after watching television for a while they may drift on to other things, or they have to reread an article because they are not taking it in. The problem here is not that they cannot understand what they are viewing or reading, but that they cannot sustain the mental effort.

Selective attention

'I can't concentrate on my coursework
if there are noises in the house.'
'I can't follow what someone is saying in a crowded pub.'

Poor selective attention refers to having difficulty concentrating on a task and ignoring distractions. We deal with many tasks surrounded by distractions. When shopping, there may be bustle and noise in the shop; while studying there may be a radio on in a nearby room. As well as being able to concentrate on things, we also need to be able to filter out or ignore these distractions. This skill is called selective attention, and refers to the ability to concentrate selectively on one item while ignoring another. After head injury, this key ability may be affected, so that it is hard to ignore distractions.

Divided attention

'I can't keep my mind on the cooking if someone talks to me.'
'I can't take in what the teacher is saying, and make notes at the same time.'

Difficulty with divided attention occurs when someone finds it hard to do two or more things at the same time. There are many situations in which we need to do several things at once – for instance, driving and talking; speaking on the telephone and writing down a message; working on equipment and listening to instructions. In these situations we have to divide or split our attention between different sources of information. This is one of the most complex attentional skills, and after head injury many people find it more difficult coping with such tasks.

Session 8

Aims of the session

1 To understand the nature of executive problems.
2 To increase awareness of the impact of executive dysfunction on everyday living.

Session outline

While many TBI survivors have some awareness of their memory and attention difficulties, fewer complain spontaneously of executive impairments – not least because a common feature of the dysexecutive syndrome is loss of insight.

Outline of executive skills

The session begins with the trainer introducing the metaphor that the brain can be thought of as being like a business run by a board of directors, at the head of which is the chief executive. An overhead (Overhead 8.1) can be used to illustrate the metaphor, with the chief executive seated at the head of a table of directors, such as the Head of Human Resources, Marketing, Finance, and so on. The trainees are then asked to consider what role the chief executive has in the company.

The trainer should elicit that the chief executive's role is to plan, organise and co-ordinate the activity of others around the table, and elsewhere within the company; to be aware of changes in the marketplace; and to be responsible for the presentation of the company to customers and competitors. The trainer or a trainee writes these roles on a flip-chart, which is divided in two, with the trainees' ideas on the left. It can be emphasised that the chief executive usually does not have a 'hands-on' role, and that although they may not be involved directly in making a product, they are nevertheless essential to the success of the company.

Next, the trainer asks the group to consider what would happen if the chief executive left and was not replaced, or could not work, perhaps through ill-health. Trainees' suggestions are added to the right half of the flip-chart, opposite the previously suggested functions. It can be pointed out that, although theoretically all the other directors should be able to continue working normally, their efforts are likely to become poorly coordinated; the identification of problems and solutions will suffer; and decision-making is likely to become erratic, impulsive or inflexible. The trainer should emphasise the fact that similar difficulties can be expected if the executive system in the brain is faulty, due to TBI. While many skills such as mathematical reasoning, reading, writing, speech and comprehension may all be intact, nevertheless, the TBI survivor may have difficulty solving problems and functioning normally. Finally, the role of the frontal lobes in underpinning executive functioning can be discussed.

Case analysis: *Mark*

The trainer then introduces the case of *Mark* (Handout 9) for the group to analyse in the same manner as *Lucy*. Two or three small groups are formed, with a trainer who acts as a facilitator. The trainees are again asked to imagine that they are Mark's doctor or therapist, and that their job is to answer each of the questions on the handout. The questions, and each group's ideas are written on a flip-chart, and a volunteer from each group is asked to feed back their views to the full group at the end of the session.

Again, particular emphasis is placed on identifying strategies that Mark could adopt to ameliorate his difficulties, drawing on previous sessions or ideas discussed in other rehabilitation groups, literature, or advice from professionals. Form 8.1 is a sample of a completed flip-chart. Following the feedback, the group is asked to consider whether Mark's situation might be improved if he followed their recommendations, and what outstanding problems remain. The aim is to help trainees identify a range of strategies which, cumulatively, might ameliorate the impact of dysexecutive impairments, and improve everyday living.

Finally, a handout (Handout 10) is provided, which summarises the material covered in the session.

Check when done

☐ 1 Recap previous session

☐ 2 Outline of executive skills: group exercise

☐ 3 Dysexecutive impairments and frontal lobe injury

☐ 4 Case analysis: *Mark*

☐ 5 Questions and answers

☐ 6 Handouts circulated (Handouts 9 and 10)

Session evaluation

(review issues/topics arising, type and quality of group interaction, suitability of material, topics requiring further review)

Trainees' progress

(note individual trainee's participation in session; comprehension and retention of material; emotional response to material and to other trainees; need for additional individual education or support)

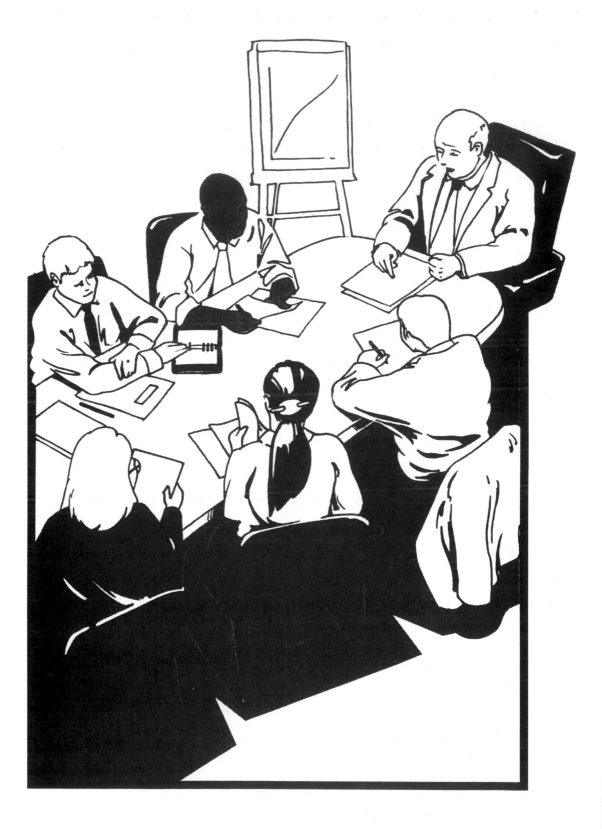

CASE STUDY: MARK

Before his head injury, Mark was a college student who achieved good grades on his computer course. Afterwards, he did not want to return to college immediately, although this remained his aim.

His father said that Mark spent his time on his computer, apparently working diligently at programmes to get himself back to his old standard. He was at the computer most days, and he frequently read computer magazines. However, as the months went by, his father began to notice that none of this activity seemed to lead anywhere, or be productive. Often, Mark was not really studying, but playing computer games. Mark would start a task with enthusiasm, but then lose interest and give up. His father also noticed that on other occasions he had difficulty getting started on chores, and he was easily muddled, although he did not always seem to appreciate he was having difficulties.

On one occasion, Mark tried to help his father strip down and clean a motorbike, something he had done many times before his injury. However, he became confused about how to go about it and which tools to use, and he put the components back together in the wrong order, and then had to dismantle them to correct what he had done. He tried to reassemble the bike in the same incorrect manner several times, but could not figure out what he was doing wrong. As a result, he became extremely frustrated, threw down his tools and gave up.

What are…
◆ *The key difficulties Mark is experiencing?*
◆ *The effects on his daily life?*
◆ *The potential causes of his problems?*
◆ *The factors that make his situation more difficult?*
◆ *The factors that would help him handle the situation better?*

CASE ANALYSIS: MARK

What are...

The key difficulties Mark is experiencing?

Does things, but not very productive

Difficulty getting started (difficulty initiating)

Easily confused and muddled

Repeats the same mistakes (gets stuck in a groove)

The effects on his daily life?

Doesn't seem to get going with his studies

Not getting back to college

Can't cope with things like he did before his injury (eg, motorbike)

Gets annoyed

The potential causes of his problems?

Head injury – sounds like he's got frontal lobe/dysexecutive problems

The factors that make his situation more difficult?

Doesn't know what he's doing wrong (lacks insight?), and makes him frustrated

The factors that would help him handle the situation better?

Needs to understand his problems better – go to Headway, read books/pamphlets on head injury

Ask for help – go for rehab

Keep checklists to guide him through tasks (eg, his motorbike)

Talk to his father (and listen)

Start getting busy one step at a time (eg, go to a club, start seeing friends)

EXECUTIVE PROBLEMS AFTER TRAUMATIC BRAIN INJURY (TBI)

Traumatic brain injury (TBI) can affect what are called our executive skills, resulting in *dysexecutive impairments*. What are executive skills? The brain can be thought of as being like a company, which consists of a range of different departments and sites, each of which complete different tasks. At the head of the company is a Chief Executive, or Chairperson, who directs the activities of the various heads of departments, who in turn influence the activities of people on the shop-floor. The frontal lobes of the brain are thought to have a similar role, in that they are important for planning and organising behaviour; making judgements about how to solve problems; and helping us stop or inhibit certain activities.

Damage to the frontal lobes can result in impairments to these executive skills. After a head injury, someone may become highly *impulsive*, and act or say things on the spur of the moment. Sometimes they behave in an embarrassing way and, for instance, they may be rude or abrupt, or make inappropriate comments. Sometimes they may become quite *rigid* and *inflexible*, and want to stick to fixed routines. They may have difficulty *planning ahead* or *organising* themselves, so that they become disorganised and chaotic.

A particular complication is that not uncommonly, people with dysexecutive difficulties *lack insight* into their difficulties. This can be apparent when a relative is asked for their opinion, and they describe more problems than were acknowledged by the TBI survivor. Loss of insight or

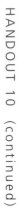
EXECUTIVE PROBLEMS AFTER TRAUMATIC BRAIN INJURY (TBI)

self-awareness is usually due to brain damage, in the same way that forgetfulness or loss of concentration may occur after head injury. One of the consequences is that a TBI survivor may be reluctant to take part in rehabilitation for problems they do not recognise or do not view as being particularly serious.

On the surface, people with dysexecutive difficulties can seem quite unaffected by their head injury. They may have many intact abilities that allow them to interact well, at least at a casual meeting. They may have essentially normal speech, reading, writing and mathematical skills, and on tests of reasoning they may perform well. However, just as a company can have all the components for success, but nevertheless fail without a Chief Executive, so a person with a head injury may have difficulty harnessing their skills to cope with the demands placed upon them.

In the first instance, dysexecutive problems can be overcome by becoming aware of their impact on daily living. It can be helpful to read about TBI, and to meet other head-injured people to obtain a different perspective. Joining a support group can be helpful. Family and friends can be a useful source of feedback to raise self-awareness. Adopting some straightforward strategies can also help reduce some dysexecutive problems; for instance, establishing a structured week of routine activities can reduce disorganisation; checklists can be used with complex tasks; and a diary system can enhance organisational skills.

Session 9

Aims of the session

Session outline

Causes of emotional problems

Overcoming emotional difficulties

Case analysis: *Jake*

Aims of the session

1 To identify the different kinds of post-TBI emotional problems.

2 To examine the potential causes of emotional problems.

3 To explore strategies to aid emotional control.

Session outline

The session begins with the trainer stating that after TBI many people experience not only cognitive problems, such as poor memory and concentration, but emotional and behavioural changes as well. Trainees are asked individually to spend a few minutes generating a list of emotional problems they have experienced, which are then entered in the first column of a self-rating form (Handout 11). The lists are then pooled, and recorded on a flip-chart. The final list may be lengthy, and include complaints such as:

Depression

Irritability

Fearfulness

Low self-esteem

Anxiety

Anger

Mood swings

Aggression

Invariably the changes volunteered are uniformly negative, although depending on the composition of the group, some trainees may think of positive changes, such as *value family more, less driven, appreciate life.*

Causes of emotional problems

The group are then asked to list some of the causes they have identified for these problems – in the middle column of the self-assessment form (Handout 11) – and these ideas are also then pooled on a flip-chart. Responses may include:

Head injury
Damage to frontal lobes
Lost job
Noise
Family don't understand
Lost friends, alone
Nothing to do
Situation too demanding – eg, too many people
Tiredness
No money
Bored

The next step is to group these possible causes under different headings:

Physical
Psychological
Social
Environmental

Physical factors might include frontal lobe damage, pain, or poor vision. Psychological factors include personal feelings, such as boredom or loss. Social factors include the response of the family, friends or employers. Environmental factors include noise, heat, physical surroundings, and so on. Flexibility is required in classifying these ideas, as necessarily some will not be grouped readily in this manner.

Overcoming emotional difficulties

Finally, the trainer asks the group to brainstorm ideas and strategies that can be adopted to address these different causes. These ideas should be listed in the final column of the self-assessment form (Handout 11); fed back to the whole group, and recorded on a flip-chart. The aim is to highlight that emotional problems often have many different causes – the direct effects of brain trauma being only one. In addition, while neurological damage may not be amenable to change, many other potential causes can be addressed by the TBI survivor, either independently, or with the help of family, friends and the rehabilitation staff.

Case analysis: *Jake*

The group then breaks into two or three small groups to analyse the case of *Jake* (Handout 12). The group is asked to approach the task in the same manner as *Lucy* and *Mark*: that is, they have to imagine they are his treating clinicians, and address each of the questions listed below the case. Trainees are asked to consider particularly the possible causes of Jake's difficulties, and what might be done to overcome them. As in previous sessions, the small groups are asked to record their ideas on a flip-chart, and a trainee provides feedback to the full group at the end of the session. A completed sample is shown in Form 9.1. Finally, Handout 13, which summarises some of the issues covered in the session, is circulated for home reading.

Check when done

- ☐ 1 Recap previous session
- ☐ 2 Self-assessment of emotional state
- ☐ 3 Causes of emotional problems: group exercise
- ☐ 4 Overcoming emotional difficulties
- ☐ 5 Case analysis: *Jake*
- ☐ 6 Questions and answers
- ☐ 7 Handouts circulated (Handouts 11–13)

Session evaluation

(review issues/topics arising, type and quality of group interaction, suitability of material, topics requiring further review)

Trainees' progress

(note individual trainee's participation in session; comprehension and retention of material; emotional response to material and to other trainees; need for additional individual education or support)

EMOTIONAL PROBLEMS: SELF-ASSESSMENT FORM

Emotional problems: Write below any emotional difficulties you have experienced since your head injury (eg, feeling low, bored, irritable, etc)	Causes: List the causes of problems you have experienced (eg, alcohol makes me short-tempered, noise, not working, etc)	Solutions: Write below the strategies or solutions you could use to overcome your emotional problems (eg, pace myself, practise relaxation exercises, take medication, etc)

CASE STUDY: JAKE

Jake – 36 years of age – was a high-flying career man running his own advertising business. One evening, he was attacked by two men in a car park and his wallet was stolen. He suffered serious injuries and was admitted to hospital, and remained in a coma for a day. Afterwards, for about 3 weeks, he was confused and did not seem to be taking things in properly. He then returned home to his family with no physical problems, apart from severe headaches.

A few weeks later, Jake made the decision to return to work. Soon difficulties began to surface. When staff were a few minutes late arriving at work, he talked down to them. On the telephone he was abrupt with customers who were slow to make decisions. With his staff he was extremely impatient if deadlines were not met. He felt bitter about the attack, which was unprovoked, and found himself dwelling on it.

At home Jake was even more demanding. He insisted that meals were ready on time. He could not tolerate the noise of his children playing, or the mess they left afterwards. After a few drinks he was particularly quick-tempered, and also when he was tired at the end of the day. His wife felt that she had constantly to check what she said, in case she upset him, and she said that living with him was like walking on eggshells.

What are…
◆ *The key difficulties Jake is experiencing?*
◆ *The effects on his daily life?*
◆ *The potential causes of his problems?*
◆ *The factors that make his situation more difficult?*
◆ *The factors that would help him handle the situation better?*

CASE ANALYSIS: JAKE

What are...

The key difficulties Jake is experiencing?

Temper

Intolerant, impatient and abrupt

Dwells on the attack

The effects on his daily life?

Not getting on with colleagues, wife, customers

Doesn't enjoy being with his children

The potential causes of his problems?

Serious head injury – he was in a coma for a day, and post-traumatic amnesia for three weeks

The factors that make his situation more difficult?

Returned to work after a few weeks – too soon, and not realistic

Bitterness

Noise

Tiredness

Alcohol

Wife giving in to him probably doesn't help in the long run

The factors that would help him handle the situation better?

He needs rehabilitation

Medication

Relaxation exercises

Breathing exercises

Avoid alcohol

Have regular rests – pace himself

Take time off work/go part-time

Talk to wife

Counselling for bitterness

Learn about TBI – join a group, see GP

Slow down – recovery will take time

Traumatic brain injury (TBI) may affect not only a person's cognitive abilities, but also their emotional wellbeing. Although there is often considerable variation from one person to another, many people experience changes in their personality, behaviour and emotional control.

Anxiety and depression

It is perhaps not surprising that after TBI many people experience feelings of despondency and anxiety. TBI can bring about profound changes, such as unemployment and resulting financial worries, and the future can suddenly become uncertain. Forgetfulness and poor concentration can undermine confidence and cause people to worry about their safety. They may repeatedly check appliances, or worry about the possibility of having an epileptic seizure. TBI can bring about many losses, such as the loss of a job, health, fitness, and cognitive skills. These social, cognitive and physical losses can cause a period of mourning, not unlike that following a bereavement.

Problems with anxiety and depression can be helped in a number of ways. Discussing concerns with either a family member or a rehabilitation counsellor can help. Sometimes medication is useful, and a combination of medication and counselling can be particularly effective. Practical steps to develop new roles to replace old ones are important: for instance, retraining for a new job, or starting college courses or voluntary work may all be constructive.

Irritability and anger

A tendency to be irritable and short-tempered is not uncommon after TBI. Problems that previously would have caused no particular upset may precipitate an outburst of frustration and anger. Noise or untidiness, a chance remark or misunderstanding, or some other minor infringement, can cause a TBI survivor to vent their anger.

Often frustration is expressed only verbally, although occasionally they may hit or throw objects, or threaten others. These mood swings can be caused by frustration with cognitive, social, financial or other problems, but they can also be due to the trauma to the brain and, in particular, damage to the frontal lobes, which are known to be important in regulating self-control and restraint.

Dealing with these problems involves becoming aware of the triggers for these feelings. Noise, tiredness, pain, inactivity, long hours and alcohol, are all examples of potential causes. The next step is to take practical steps to deal with these triggers; for instance, avoiding alcohol, taking rests, developing new activities. Other methods that reduce irritability, such as relaxation or breathing exercises, yoga, and medication may also be useful.

Disinhibition and poor motivation

Damage to the frontal lobes can cause disinhibition, so that a person behaves in inappropriate or embarrassing ways. Such behaviour includes being overfamiliar or indiscreet; referring to personal matters in front of others; touching, or standing too close; talking loudly, or dressing oddly. Invariably the head-injured person is not fully aware of such problems, and consequently it can be hard to change. In this situation, feedback from others is important to become aware of such behaviour. Some people lose interest and motivation. They may do relatively little, and neglect activities that they previously enjoyed. Taking on a small range of activities, and gradually building them up over time is a useful way of kindling interest and motivation. It can be helpful to draw up a list of activities to complete, and enter them in a diary or weekly schedule that specifies when and for how long each will be completed. When done, the task can be ticked off, and with time, the number of activities gradually expanded.

Session 10

Aims of the session

> 1 To examine the relationships between cognitive, emotional and social problems.
> 2 To help trainees prepare their personal presentations.

Session outline

The session begins with the trainer pointing out that the cognitive and emotional issues that have been explored in previous sessions rarely occur in isolation, and more commonly they coexist. For instance, many people have not only memory and attentional difficulties, but also emotional problems, such as feelings of anxiety and depression. Such problems often interact: for instance, forgetfulness may cause frustration and irritability, which in turn makes it difficult to concentrate and take things in, so worsening the forgetfulness. As a result, a problem in one area can affect a person's ability to function in another, and sets up a downward cycle of problems from which it is difficult to escape. Becoming aware of how problems interact can be important in learning to overcome them; and by addressing each difficulty in turn, it may be possible to make progress.

Understanding complex problems

The group is then asked to volunteer examples of similar interactions from their own experience. If necessary, trainees should be prompted by asking if they have had a problem which seemed to get out of hand, or found themselves in a downward spiral where one difficulty led to another. These problems are shared and discussed by the group, and written on a flip-chart to illustrate the complexity of such interactions. They may include:

'Can't concentrate if I'm annoyed.'
'I can't think straight and concentrate in shops if there's a queue behind me.'
'If I'm worried, my mind goes blank, and that makes me more worried.'
'If too many people are talking, I can't take it in, and I get worked up.'
'When I'm low, I can't remember things properly,
which gets me more frustrated.'

Case analysis: *Greg*

The group are then introduced to *Greg* (Handout 14), in the same manner as previously, except that Greg's case focuses not only on isolated cognitive, emotional or social problems, but on a number of these issues, which makes analysis of his difficulties more complicated. The trainees are again asked to break into small groups to address the questions following the case, and each group's ideas are fed back to the full group, as before. Particular emphasis should be placed on understanding the interactions between different problems, and the practical steps that could be taken to overcome Greg's difficulties. The intention is to provide trainees with more practice at looking at TBI-related problems, and thinking in greater depth and detail about the full range of strategies that might ameliorate these difficulties. A completed sample analysis is provided in Form 10.1.

Preparing for personal presentations

The trainer then circulates the form *Acquired Brain Injury: Self-Assessment* (Handout 15), and discusses the aims of the final two sessions of the group. These are given over to personal presentations, in which trainees present themselves to the group. The presentation is intended to review the cause and effects of their injuries, and the strategies and techniques they intend to use to aid their recovery. The presentations should last about 10 minutes, followed by five minutes of feedback and discussion by the whole group. It is stressed that participation is voluntary, although it is hoped that by this stage in the course, all trainees will feel comfortable completing the exercise with the group. The aims of the presentations are, first, to help trainees arrive at an accurate understanding of their injuries and associated difficulties; and second, to clarify their rehabilitation plan to deal with their difficulties both currently and following completion of the group.

To help prepare their presentations, trainees are asked to work through and complete Handout 15 *Self Assessment: Acquired Brain Injury*, which is intended to condense information applicable to themselves, and discussed in previous sessions. Trainees should be encouraged to draw on a range of sources, such as the opinions of other trainees, rehabilitation staff, relatives and friends, information contained in hospital records, as well as the results of neuropsychological tests, brain scans, medico-legal reports, and outside reading. Information relating to strategies to overcome problems will invariably draw on work completed in other rehabilitation groups and individual sessions. Although the form can be started in the session, it is not possible to complete it quickly, and most people will need to meet with a member of the rehabilitation team outside the group for assistance with preparing their talk. For some trainees, their presentation may involve simply reading through the form; others may prefer to rewrite the material and present it in a quite different format. The order of presentations for the next two sessions should be agreed, with no more than four in each session.

Check when done

☐ 1 Recap previous session

☐ 2 Understanding interactions between cognitive, emotional and social problems: group exercise

☐ 3 Case analysis: *Greg*

☐ 4 Discussion of personal presentation, and circulation of self-assessment form

☐ 5 Handouts circulated (Handouts 14 and 15)

Session evaluation

(review issues/topics arising, type and quality of group interaction, suitability of material, topics requiring further review)

Trainees' progress

(note individual trainee's participation in session; comprehension and retention of material; emotional response to material and to other trainees; need for additional individual education or support)

CASE STUDY: GREG

Greg had an accident at work. He tripped and fell 6 metres from scaffolding. He suffered a skull fracture, and he was unconscious for two days, and confused and disoriented for a further four or five days. As well as a head injury, he suffered injuries to his spine and right shoulder. He became quite forgetful and, for instance, he would mislay his keys or wallet, and sometimes forget arrangements to meet people. His speech was a little slurred, and he had difficulty choosing the right word, particularly when tired. He suffered from dizziness and his balance was quite poor.

Before his accident, Greg had always been a little quiet and he was never inclined to mix. Afterwards, he became anxious about his balance, and he was reluctant to go out in case he fell, although he had never done so. He lacked confidence and was easily flustered by people. In company, he became nervous and had difficulty thinking clearly, which made him feel all the more anxious. He tended to tire easily during the day, and when he became fatigued he was easily annoyed.

Greg did not return to work, and consequently he had little to do, and spent a lot of time at home worrying about bills and the future. He had pain in his back and shoulder, which also made him irritable. As a result, his confidence declined and he became despondent.

Occasionally, Greg tried to improve things and, for instance, he enrolled on a full range of courses throughout the week. However, he found it hard to cope with the demands of a week's studies, and after a month he gave up. He eventually concluded that if he could not do things as he had done before his accident, he would not do them at all.

What are…
◆ *The key difficulties Greg is experiencing?*
◆ *The effects on his daily life?*
◆ *The potential causes of his problems?*
◆ *The factors that make his situation more difficult?*
◆ *The factors that would help him handle the situation better?*

CASE ANALYSIS: GREG

What are...

The key difficulties Greg is experiencing?

Forgetfulness and slurred speech

Difficulty choosing words

Anxious – about balance and falling

Lacks confidence

Nervous in company and gets flustered

The effects on his daily life?

Not working

Doesn't like to go out because of balance

Doesn't want to mix

Can't cope with studying

The potential causes of his problems?

Serious head injury – unconscious for two days and PTA for 4–5 days, and skull fracture. May have had some frontal lobe damage, because his personality is different, and temporal lobe damage because he is forgetful.

The factors that make his situation more difficult?

Tiredness and pain

Quiet person before, and perhaps more likely to be anxious afterwards (?)

Worries a lot – worrying won't change situation

His response to his problems – says he won't do anything if he can't be like he was before

The factors that would help him handle the situation better?

Cognitive problems

Use memory aids (eg, diary, planners, wallchart, calendar)

Establish a daily routine so he is less likely to forget things

Put keys and wallet in a regular place

Emotional problems

Practise relaxation exercises

Take medication

Counselling

Go to drop-in centre/self-help group, and build up his hours gradually – being inactive allows him to focus on the pain

Take rests and pace himself to cope with fatigue

Discuss finances with social worker/advice service

ACQUIRED BRAIN INJURY: SELF-ASSESSMENT

Name _____

Date _____ Date of injury _____

How did the injury occur? (eg, road traffic accident, fall, assault, industrial injury, sporting accident)

How severe was the injury? (eg, how long unconscious, length of post-traumatic amnesia, presence/absence of skull fracture, bleed inside skull)

What area(s) of the brain were affected? (eg, left/right hemispheres, frontal, temporal, parietal, occipital lobes)

What cognitive problems do you have now? (eg, forget conversations or shopping, difficulty concentrating when reading or studying, difficulty solving problems, finding words, spelling, dealing with figures, etc)

1 _____

2 _____

3 _____

4 _____

5 _____

What cognitive strengths do you have? (eg, list those abilities and skills that have not been affected by your head injury)

1 _____

2 _____

3 _____

4 _____

5 _____

What emotional/behavioural problems do you have now? (eg, feel low and depressed; tend to be irritable and easily annoyed; bored; worry a lot; mood swings quickly for no reason; can be impulsive and act without thinking; say the wrong thing, etc)

1 _____

2 _____

3 _____

4 _____

5 _____

What emotional/character strengths do you have? (eg, good sense of humour; like being with people; good company with people I know; have a circle of friends, etc)

1 _____

2 _____

3 _____

4 _____

5 _____

ACQUIRED BRAIN INJURY: SELF-ASSESSMENT

What strategies are you using to deal with your cognitive problems? (eg, use diary or daily planner, dictaphone, personal organiser, message board; follow a structured routine; pace myself – work for short periods, take regular rests, avoid late nights; use a pill reminder, etc)

1 _____

2 _____

3 _____

4 _____

5 _____

What strategies are you using to deal with your emotional problems? (eg, practise relaxation exercises; take medication; attend a support group; talk more to family and friends; avoid alcohol/drugs; take regular rests; meditate; practise breathing exercises; ask for feedback from others, etc)

1 _____

2 _____

3 _____

4 _____

5 _____

What are your rehabilitation goals for the next month? (eg, practise diary use; restart old hobby; go to drop-in centre; go to gym; visit job centre; prepare weekly meal; shop weekly, etc)

ACQUIRED BRAIN INJURY: SELF-ASSESSMENT

What are your rehabilitation goals for the next six months? (eg, go to college; start voluntary work; change accommodation; return to work; learn word-processing, etc)

Sessions 11 and 12

Aim of the session

> **1 To allow trainees to make their personal presentations, and review their injuries and current and future rehabilitation goals.**

Session outline

The trainer begins by dealing with any queries or issues that arise, before moving on to the personal presentations.

Trainees' personal presentations

Trainees can move to a central chair, or speak from their existing position. The format of each presentation should be agreed before the meeting, in consultation with a trainer. Some trainees may decide to read aloud the details on their self-assessment form (Handout 15), whereas others will adopt a different format. The presentations are not intended to be formal occasions, and with some trainees there may be a good deal of humour and interaction. An important function of the presentation, however, is for each trainee to have arrived at an accurate understanding of their injuries and resulting difficulties, and to have a clear, self-directed plan to overcome those difficulties. The quality of the presentation is therefore far less important than the degree to which these goals are achieved.

When the trainee has finished, the group are asked to provide feedback – for instance, suggesting additional strategies or approaches that the trainee might consider. The exercise is intended to be a supportive and encouraging experience, and to mark the conclusion of the course, rather than explore or address new issues.

Following the presentations, it may be helpful for the trainers to summarise reflectively what appear to be common themes and issues that have emerged, and the group may want to discuss these further. The trainers have a number of important roles that amplify their approach during previous sessions. These include:

◆ Confirming accurate understanding
◆ Endorsing insightful comments
◆ Supporting constructive plans
◆ Encouraging self-efficacy and responsibility
◆ Stressing the importance of personal motivation.

The trainers may cue trainees if they have overlooked instances of progress, or strategies that might be of use. When a trainee is uncertain about their progress, goals or strategies, the trainers may ask the group for feedback. Plans that are realistic and pragmatic should be attended to and endorsed, to encourage generalisation. The trainers should particularly encourage and stress the importance of personal responsibility and motivation for maintaining strategies after completion of the programme.

Check when done

☐ 1 Recap previous session

☐ 2 Trainees' personal presentations

☐ 3 Group feedback following presentations

Session evaluation

(review issues/topics arising, type and quality of group interaction, suitability of material, topics requiring further review)

Trainees' progress

(note individual trainee's participation in session; comprehension and retention of material; emotional response to material and to other trainees; need for additional individual education or support)

Bibliography

Ben-Yishay Y, 1996, 'Reflections on the Evolution of the Therapeutic Milieu Concept', *Neuropsychological Rehabilitation* 6, pp327–43.

British Society of Rehabilitation Medicine, 1998, *Rehabilitation after Traumatic Brain Injury: A Working Party Report of the British Society of Rehabilitation Medicine*, British Society of Rehabilitation Medicine, London.

Brooks N, McKinlay W, Symington C, Beattie A & Campsie L, 1987a, 'Return to work within the first seven years of head injury', *Brain Injury* 1, pp5–19.

Brooks N, McKinlay W, Symington C, Beattie A & Campsie L, 1987b, 'The effects of severe head injury on patient and relative within seven years of injury', *Journal of Head Trauma Rehabilitation* 2, pp1–13.

Christensen AL, Caetano C & Rasmussen G, 1996, 'Psychosocial outcome after an intensive neuropsychologically oriented day program: contributing program variables', Uzzell BP & Stonnington HH (eds), *Recovery after Traumatic Brain Injury*, Lawrence Erlbaum, New Jersey.

Giacino JT & Cicerone KD, 1998, 'Varieties of deficit unawareness after brain injury', *Journal of Head Trauma Rehabilitation* 13, pp1–15.

McMillan TM & Sparkes C, 1999, 'Goal Planning and Neurorehabilitation: The Wolfson Neurorehabilitation Centre Approach', *Neuropsychological Rehabilitation* 9, pp241–51.

Ponsford JL, 1995, *Traumatic Brain Injury: Rehabilitation for Everyday Adaptive Living*, Lawrence Erlbaum, Hove.

Ponsford JL, Olver JH & Curran C, 1996, 'Outcome following traumatic brain injury; an Australian study', Uzzell BP & Stonnington HH (eds), *Recovery after Traumatic Brain Injury*, Lawrence Erlbaum, New Jersey.

Prigatano GP, 1991, 'Disturbance of self-awareness of deficit after traumatic brain injury', Prigatano GP & Schacter DI (eds), *Awareness of Deficits after Brain Injury: Clinical and Theoretical Issues*, Oxford University Press, New York.

Prigatano GP, 1997, 'The problem of impaired self-awareness in neuropsychological rehabilitation', Carrion L (ed), *Neuropsychological Rehabilitation: Fundamentals, Innovations and Directions*, GR Press/St Lucie Press, Florida.

Prigatano GP & Weinstein EA, 1996, 'Edwin A Weinstein's contributions to neuropsychological rehabilitation', *Neuropsychological Rehabilitation* 6, pp305–26.

Sherer M, Bergloff P, Levin E, High WM, Oden KE & Nick TG, 1998, 'Impaired awareness and employment outcome after traumatic brain injury', *Journal of Head Trauma Rehabilitation* 13, pp52–61.

Sohlberg MM, Johansen A, Geyer S & Hoornbeek S, 1994, *A Manual for Teaching Patients to Use Compensatory Memory Systems*, Association for Neuropsychological Research and Development, Puyallup.

Sohlberg MM & Mateer CA, 1987, 'Effectiveness of an attention-training program', *Journal of Clinical and Experimental Neuropsychology* 9, pp117–30.

Sohlberg MM & Raskin SA, 1996, 'Principles of generalisation applied to attention and memory interventions', *Journal of Head Trauma Rehabilitation* 11, pp65–78.

Tobbell J & Burns J, 1997, *GAS: Goal Attainment Scaling for People with Learning Disabilities*, Speechmark Publishing/Winslow Press, Bicester.

van den Broek MD, 1999, 'Cognitive rehabilitation and traumatic brain injury', *Reviews in Clinical Gerontology* 9, pp257–64.

Wesolowski MD & Zencius AH, 1994, *A Practical Guide to Head Injury Rehabilitation: A Focus on Postacute Residential Treatment*, Plenum, New York.

Related Titles Published by Speechmark

Head Injury
A Practical Guide

Trevor Powell
Foreword by Diana, Princess of Wales

This excellent book provide professionals, families and carers with a practical and down-to-earth guide to the hidden psychological, social, behavioural and emotional problems caused by head injury.

Written in jargon-free style, it addresses the medical problems, rehabilitation and adjustment of individuals and families to the realities of life after head injury.

Sourcebooks for Neurodisability

Sourcebook for Adults with Profound Communication Difficulties

Fiona Sugden-Best

Clients who have limited motor control, with a reliance on a yes/no response and/or eye pointing are the target audience for this sourcebook. Its emphasis is on informing carers and giving them the support to work independently with their dependant. Overall, this practical book demonstrates that there is still a lot of work and assessment that can be done to support this type of caseload.

Contents include:

- *Oromotor Exercises*: for face, lip, tongue, jaw and palate, photocopiable exercises in large format with pictures to aid clients to work independently. There is also a desensitisation programme for the face and oral area.

- *Articulation Sheets*: for each sound in initial, medial and final positions as appropriate.

- *Language Assessments*: includes a sensory stimulation programme, a yes/no screen and an initial language screen. The assessments are designed so clients require only a reliable yes/no response to answer syntactically complex questions.

- *AAC*: a screening form to assess clients who are able to eye-point and assess the potential of this skill to use an AAC device.

- *Handouts, Questionnaires & Breathing*: this includes sheets for carers to explain the type of communication difficulty their dependent is experiencing.

Sourcebook for Assessing & Maintaining Communication

Fiona Sugden-Best

The second volume in the series *Sourcebooks for Neurodisability*, this book is aimed at clients who have some, even if limited, motor control to enable hand pointing. Contains many photocopiable exercises that can be handed to clients and carers to work on independently, with record sheets that can be easily filled in. The sourcebook contains:

- *Oromotor Exercises*: laid out in a clear format, with illustrations, enabling clients to work independently. Record sheets to fill in on a daily basis.

- *Articulation Sheets*: speech sounds, including consonant clusters, of multi-syllabic words and tongue twisters. Phrases of syllabic length are also included.

- *Language Assessments & Screens*: for those reliant at a high level on hand pointing alone.

- *AAC*: screen with alphabet charts for direct access.

- *Handouts*: to give to the client for awareness of their specific communication difficulties.

- *Questionnaires & Breathing and Voice Parameters*: includes breathing exercises and sheets relating to relaxation and posture, pitch, intonation and resonance exercises all to give to the client. Photocopiable record sheets for the client to fill in on how they rate their speech are also included.

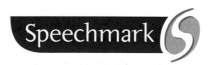

**Telford Road • Bicester
Oxon • OX26 4LQ • UK**
Tel: **(01869) 244644**
Fax: **(01869) 320040**
www.winslow-press.co.uk